Abraxxzas

The Tomato Chronicles

Unveiling Nature's Red Treasure

Contents

   1.

   2.

   3.

   4.

   5.

   6.

   7.

8.

9.

10.

11.

12.

13.

14.

15.

16.

17.

18.

19.

20.

21.

22.

23.

1

Chapter 1

2

THE TOMATO CHRONICLES

3

Unveiling Nature's Red Treasure

4

Chapter 1: A Brief History of Tomatoes

Tomatoes, the juicy red fruits we enjoy today, have a rich and fascinating history that spans centuries and continents. Native to the Andes region of South America, specifically Peru, Ecuador, and Bolivia, tomatoes have a lineage that dates back thousands of years.

1.1 Early Cultivation:

Tomatoes were first cultivated by indigenous peoples in these regions as early as 500 BC. The earliest evidence of tomato cultivation comes from ancient pottery depicting tomatoes found in Peru. These early tomatoes were small and likely bore little resemblance to the plump, juicy fruits we are familiar with today.

1.2 Introduction to Europe:

The Spanish conquistadors are credited with introducing tomatoes to Europe in the 16th century after their conquests in Central and South America. However, early European encounters with tomatoes were met with suspicion and skepticism. Initially, tomatoes were grown as ornamental plants rather than for consumption, as they were mistakenly believed to be poisonous due to their resemblance to the deadly nightshade plant.

1.3 Tomatoes Conquer Italy:

Despite initial reservations, tomatoes gradually gained popularity in Europe, particularly in Italy. By the 17th century, tomatoes had become a staple ingredient in Italian cuisine, featuring prominently in dishes such as pasta sauces and pizzas. The discovery of the tomato's culinary potential revolutionized Italian cooking and paved the way for tomatoes to become an essential ingredient in cuisines around the world.

1.4 Spread Across the Globe:

From Italy, the cultivation and consumption of tomatoes spread throughout Europe and beyond. In the 18th century, tomatoes made their way to North America, where they were embraced by Native American tribes and eventually became a staple in American cuisine. Today, tomatoes are cultivated on every continent except Antarctica, with hundreds of varieties grown worldwide.

1.5 Modern Cultivation and Varieties:

Modern tomato cultivation has led to the development of numerous tomato varieties, each with its unique flavor, size, and color. From the classic beefsteak tomato to cherry tomatoes, heirloom varieties, and more, there is a tomato to suit every taste and culinary preference.

1.6 Conclusion:

The history of tomatoes is a testament to the resilience and adaptability of this humble fruit. From its humble beginnings in the Andes Mountains to its status as a global culinary staple, the tomato's journey is a story of exploration, innovation, and cultural exchange. As we continue to uncover the health benefits and culinary possibilities of tomatoes, we honor their rich history and celebrate their place as nature's red treasure.

5

Chapter 2: The Botanical Wonders of Tomatoes

Tomatoes (Solanum lycopersicum) are not just delicious and versatile; they are also fascinating from a botanical perspective. In this chapter, we'll delve into the unique botanical characteristics of tomatoes and explore what makes them such remarkable plants.

2.1 Taxonomy and Classification:

Tomatoes belong to the Solanaceae family, which includes other well-known plants such as potatoes, eggplants, and peppers. Within the Solanaceae family, tomatoes belong to the Solanum genus, along with thousands of other species. The scientific name for tomatoes, Solanum lycopersicum, reflects their botanical classification.

2.2 Growth Habit and Structure:

Tomatoes are herbaceous plants that can grow as annuals or perennials, depending on the climate and growing conditions. They are typically grown as annuals in temperate regions, where they complete their life cycle within a single growing season. Tomatoes are characterized by their sprawling growth habit, with long, vining stems that require support for optimal growth. The leaves of tomato plants are pinnately compound, consisting of multiple leaflets arranged along a central stem. The flowers of tomato plants are small and yellow, typically borne in clusters.

2.3 Fruit Development:

One of the most distinctive features of tomatoes is their fruit, which botanically speaking, is classified as a berry. Tomatoes develop from the ovary of the flower and undergo a process called parthenocarpy, which means they can produce fruit without fertilization. The development of tomatoes involves several stages, beginning with pollination and fertilization of the flower, followed by fruit set and maturation. As the fruit matures, it changes color from green to red (or other colors depending on the variety) and undergoes biochemical changes that contribute to its flavor, aroma, and nutritional content.

2.4 Genetic Diversity:

Tomatoes exhibit a remarkable degree of genetic diversity, with thousands of cultivated varieties available worldwide. This genetic diversity has been shaped by centuries of selective breeding by farmers and breeders, resulting in tomatoes of various shapes, sizes, colors, and flavors. From classic round tomatoes to elongated plum tomatoes, cherry tomatoes, and heirloom varieties with unique traits, there is a tomato variety to suit every taste and culinary preference.

2.5 Wild Relatives and Conservation:

In addition to cultivated varieties, tomatoes also have wild relatives that grow in diverse habitats around the world. These wild relatives, known as wild tomatoes or cherry tomatoes, play a crucial role in tomato breeding programs aimed at improving disease resistance, yield, and other desirable traits. However, many wild tomato species are also threatened by habitat loss, climate change, and other factors, highlighting the importance of conservation efforts to preserve tomato genetic diversity for future generations.

2.6 Conclusion:

From their sprawling vines to their flavorful fruits and rich genetic diversity, tomatoes are truly botanical wonders. As we continue to explore and appreciate the unique characteristics of tomatoes, we gain a deeper understanding of their importance as both a culinary staple and a valuable genetic resource. In the following chapters, we will delve into the nutritional benefits, health properties, and culinary uses of tomatoes, unlocking the full potential of nature's red treasure.

6

Chapter 3: Tomatoes Around the World

Tomatoes have become a ubiquitous ingredient in cuisines around the world, beloved for their versatility, flavor, and nutritional value. In this chapter, we will embark on a journey to explore how tomatoes are cultivated, prepared, and enjoyed in different regions and cultures across the globe.

3.1 The Mediterranean:

In the Mediterranean region, tomatoes hold a central place in culinary traditions, particularly in countries such as Italy, Greece, Spain, and France. Italian cuisine, in particular, features tomatoes in a myriad of dishes, from classic pasta sauces like marinara and arrabbiata to Caprese salads and Margherita pizzas. In Greece, tomatoes are used in salads, sauces, and stews, while Spanish cuisine showcases tomatoes in dishes like gazpacho, a refreshing cold soup made with tomatoes, peppers, onions, and other vegetables.

3.2 North America:

In North America, tomatoes are a staple ingredient in American and Mexican cuisines. In the United States, tomatoes are used in a wide range of dishes, including burgers, sandwiches, salads, and soups. Southern-style tomato dishes, such as fried green tomatoes and tomato pie, are also popular in the Southern states. In Mexico, tomatoes are essential components of dishes like salsa, guacamole, and pico de gallo, adding vibrant color and flavor to traditional Mexican cuisine.

3.3 Asia:

In Asia, tomatoes are used in diverse ways across different cuisines. In Indian cuisine, tomatoes are used as a base for curries, sauces, and chutneys, adding richness and tanginess to dishes. In Chinese cuisine, tomatoes are often stir-fried with other vegetables or used in soups and braised dishes. In Southeast Asia, tomatoes are used in salads, stir-fries, and as a garnish for noodle dishes, adding a refreshing contrast to spicy and savory flavors.

3.4 Middle East:

In the Middle East, tomatoes are integral to dishes in countries such as Lebanon, Syria, Israel, and Turkey. Tomatoes are used in dishes like tabbouleh, a refreshing salad made with parsley, bulgur wheat, tomatoes, and lemon juice. Tomatoes are also used in sauces and stews, such as the popular Turkish dish Menemen, a breakfast dish made with tomatoes, peppers, and eggs.

3.5 Africa:

In Africa, tomatoes are widely used in cuisines across the continent, from North Africa to sub-Saharan Africa. In countries like Nigeria, tomatoes are used in soups, stews, and sauces, such as the spicy tomato-based stew known as jollof rice. In North African countries like Morocco and Tunisia, tomatoes are used in tagines, couscous dishes, and salads, adding vibrant color and flavor to traditional North African cuisine.

3.6 Conclusion:

The global popularity of tomatoes is a testament to their versatility, adaptability, and universal appeal. Whether used as a base for sauces, soups, and stews or enjoyed fresh in salads and sandwiches, tomatoes play a central role in cuisines around the world. As we continue to explore the culinary diversity of tomatoes, we gain a deeper appreciation for their role as nature's red treasure, enriching dishes and delighting taste buds across continents   and   cultures.

7

Chapter 4: Nutritional Breakdown: What Makes Tomatoes Super-foods?

Tomatoes are often hailed as superfoods, and for good reason. Packed with essential nutrients and powerful antioxidants, tomatoes offer a wide array of health benefits. In this chapter, we will explore the nutritional profile of tomatoes and uncover what makes them such nutritional powerhouses.

4.1 Vitamins and Minerals:

Tomatoes are rich in essential vitamins and minerals that are vital for overall health and well-being. They are an excellent source of vitamin C, which supports immune function, skin health, and wound healing. Tomatoes also contain vitamin K, which is important for blood clotting and bone health, as well as potassium, a mineral that helps regulate blood pressure and muscle function.

4.2 Antioxidants:

One of the key reasons tomatoes are considered superfoods is their high antioxidant content. Tomatoes are particularly rich in lycopene, a powerful antioxidant that gives them their vibrant red color. Lycopene has been linked to numerous health benefits, including reducing the risk of heart disease, certain types of cancer, and age-related macular degeneration. In addition to lycopene, tomatoes contain other antioxidants such as beta-carotene, vitamin C, and vitamin E, which help protect cells from damage caused by free radicals.

4.3 Fiber:

Tomatoes are a good source of dietary fiber, which is important for digestive health and regular bowel movements. Fiber also helps regulate blood sugar levels, lower cholesterol levels, and promote feelings of fullness, making it beneficial for weight management and overall cardiovascular health. The fiber content in tomatoes comes from both soluble and insoluble fiber, which provide different health benefits.

4.4 Low in Calories:

Despite their rich nutritional profile, tomatoes are relatively low in calories, making them a great addition to a balanced diet for those looking to manage their weight or reduce calorie intake. One medium-sized tomato contains only about 25 calories, making it a satisfying and nutritious snack or ingredient in meals without adding excess calories.

4.5 Versatility in Culinary Uses:

Beyond their nutritional benefits, tomatoes are incredibly versatile in culinary applications. They can be eaten raw in salads, sandwiches, and salsas, cooked in sauces, soups, and stews, or preserved through canning, drying, or freezing for future use. The wide variety of tomato cultivars available, from beefsteak tomatoes to cherry tomatoes and heirloom varieties, ensures that there is a tomato suitable for every dish and palate.

4.6 Conclusion:

Tomatoes truly earn their status as superfoods due to their impressive nutritional profile, antioxidant content, and culinary versatility. Whether enjoyed fresh, cooked, or preserved, tomatoes offer a delicious and nutritious addition to any diet. In the following chapters, we will delve deeper into the specific health benefits of tomatoes, exploring their role in promoting heart health, preventing cancer, supporting skin health, and much more.

8

Chapter 5: Lycopene: The Mighty Antioxidant

Lycopene is a potent antioxidant found abundantly in tomatoes and other red fruits and vegetables. In this chapter, we will explore the remarkable properties of lycopene and its profound impact on health and well-being.

5.1 What is Lycopene?

Lycopene is a carotenoid pigment that gives tomatoes their vibrant red color. It is one of the most powerful antioxidants found in nature and is responsible for many of the health benefits associated with tomato consumption. While tomatoes are the primary dietary source of lycopene, it is also found in other red fruits and vegetables such as watermelon, pink grapefruit, and red bell peppers.

5.2 Antioxidant Properties:

Lycopene is a potent scavenger of free radicals, which are unstable molecules that can damage cells and contribute to chronic diseases such as cancer, heart disease, and age-related macular degeneration. By neutralizing free radicals, lycopene helps protect cells from oxidative damage and reduces inflammation, thereby supporting overall health and longevity.

5.3 Heart Health Benefits:

Numerous studies have demonstrated the beneficial effects of lycopene on heart health. Lycopene has been shown to reduce levels of LDL cholesterol, also known as "bad" cholesterol, and inhibit the oxidation of LDL cholesterol, which can lead to the formation of plaque in the arteries. By promoting healthy cholesterol levels and reducing oxidative stress, lycopene helps lower the risk of heart disease and stroke.

5.4 Cancer Prevention:

Lycopene has been extensively studied for its potential role in cancer prevention, particularly prostate cancer. Several epidemiological studies have found an inverse association between lycopene consumption and the risk of prostate cancer, with higher lycopene intake associated with a lower risk of developing the disease. Additionally, lycopene has been shown to inhibit the growth of cancer cells and induce apoptosis, or programmed cell death, in cancer cells, further supporting its role in cancer prevention.

5.5 Skin Protection:

In addition to its internal health benefits, lycopene also offers protection against UV-induced skin damage and premature aging. Studies have shown that lycopene supplementation or topical application of lycopene-containing products can help reduce sunburn, inflammation, and oxidative stress caused by UV radiation. By neutralizing free radicals and reducing inflammation, lycopene helps protect the skin from sun damage and maintain a youthful appearance.

5.6 Conclusion:

Lycopene is truly a mighty antioxidant with a wide range of health benefits. From protecting against heart disease and cancer to promoting skin health and longevity, lycopene plays a crucial role in supporting overall health and well-being. By incorporating lycopene-rich foods like tomatoes into your diet, you can harness the power of this potent antioxidant and enjoy its many health-promoting effects.

9

Chapter 6: Tomatoes and Heart Health

Heart disease remains one of the leading causes of death worldwide, making it crucial to adopt heart-healthy habits, including dietary choices. In this chapter, we'll explore the relationship between tomatoes and heart health, uncovering how this humble fruit can contribute to cardiovascular well-being.

6.1 Lowering Cholesterol Levels:

High levels of LDL cholesterol, often referred to as "bad" cholesterol, are a major risk factor for heart disease. Studies have shown that certain compounds in tomatoes, including lycopene and fiber, can help lower LDL cholesterol levels and improve overall cholesterol profiles. Lycopene, in particular, has been found to inhibit the oxidation of LDL cholesterol, which can lead to the formation of plaque in the arteries. By reducing LDL cholesterol levels and inhibiting its oxidation, tomatoes help protect against atherosclerosis and lower the risk of heart attacks and strokes.

6.2 Supporting Healthy Blood Pressure:

High blood pressure, or hypertension, is another significant risk factor for heart disease. Potassium, a mineral found abundantly in tomatoes, plays a key role in regulating blood pressure by counteracting the effects of sodium and relaxing blood vessel walls. Additionally, the nitric oxide-boosting properties of certain compounds in tomatoes, such as nitrates and antioxidants, help promote vasodilation, further supporting healthy blood pressure levels. By incorporating tomatoes into your diet, you can help maintain healthy blood pressure and reduce the risk of hypertension-related complications.

6.3 Improving Endothelial Function:

The endothelium is the inner lining of blood vessels and plays a crucial role in regulating vascular tone, blood flow, and overall cardiovascular health. Dysfunction of the endothelium, characterized by reduced nitric oxide production and increased inflammation, is a hallmark of early-stage cardiovascular disease. Studies have shown that tomatoes and tomato products, particularly those rich in lycopene and other antioxidants, can improve endothelial function by increasing nitric oxide production, reducing inflammation, and promoting vascular health. By enhancing endothelial function, tomatoes help maintain healthy blood vessel function and reduce the risk of cardiovascular events.

6.4 Reducing Oxidative Stress and Inflammation:

Oxidative stress and inflammation are key drivers of cardiovascular disease, contributing to the development and progression of atherosclerosis, hypertension, and heart failure. The antioxidant and anti-inflammatory properties of tomatoes, particularly lycopene, help combat oxidative stress and inflammation, protecting against damage to blood vessels and the heart. By neutralizing free radicals and reducing inflammatory markers, tomatoes help mitigate the underlying processes that lead to heart disease and promote overall cardiovascular health.

6.5 Conclusion:

Tomatoes are not only delicious and versatile; they are also powerful allies in the fight against heart disease. From lowering cholesterol levels and supporting healthy blood pressure to improving endothelial function and reducing oxidative stress, tomatoes offer a multitude of benefits for heart health. By incorporating tomatoes into your diet regularly, whether fresh, cooked, or in the form of sauces and soups, you can nourish your heart and enjoy the many flavors and nutrients that nature's red treasure has to offer.

10

Chapter 7: Tomatoes and Cancer Prevention

Cancer is a devastating disease that affects millions of people worldwide, making prevention a critical aspect of overall health. In this chapter, we'll explore the relationship between tomatoes and cancer prevention, uncovering the powerful compounds in tomatoes that may help reduce the risk of various types of cancer.

7.1 Lycopene and Cancer:

Lycopene, the vibrant red pigment found abundantly in tomatoes, has been extensively studied for its potential role in cancer prevention. Numerous epidemiological studies have found an inverse association between lycopene consumption and the risk of certain types of cancer, including prostate, lung, stomach, and breast cancer. Lycopene's potent antioxidant properties help neutralize free radicals and inhibit oxidative damage to DNA, which can lead to the development of cancerous cells. Additionally, lycopene has been shown to induce apoptosis, or programmed cell death, in cancer cells, further contributing to its anticancer effects.

7.2 Prostate Cancer:

Prostate cancer is the most common cancer among men worldwide, making it a significant public health concern. Several studies have suggested that lycopene may play a protective role against prostate cancer development. In a large-scale prospective study published in the Journal of the National Cancer Institute, researchers found that higher lycopene levels in the blood were associated with a lower risk of developing aggressive prostate cancer. Other studies have reported similar findings, highlighting the potential of lycopene-rich foods like tomatoes in prostate cancer prevention.

7.3 Lung Cancer:

Lung cancer is one of the leading causes of cancer-related deaths worldwide, with smoking being the primary risk factor. However, dietary factors, including fruit and vegetable consumption, may also influence lung cancer risk. Studies have shown that a high intake of lycopene-rich foods like tomatoes is associated with a reduced risk of lung cancer, particularly in non-smokers. Lycopene's antioxidant properties help protect against oxidative damage to lung tissue caused by environmental toxins and carcinogens, thereby reducing the risk of lung cancer development.

7.4 Stomach Cancer:

Stomach cancer, also known as gastric cancer, is a significant global health burden, particularly in countries with high rates of infection with the bacterium Helicobacter pylori and low consumption of fruits and vegetables. Studies have suggested that lycopene may help protect against stomach cancer by inhibiting the growth of cancer cells and reducing inflammation in the gastric mucosa. Additionally, lycopene's antioxidant properties help neutralize reactive oxygen species (ROS) and prevent DNA damage in stomach cells, further reducing the risk of cancer development.

7.5 Breast Cancer:

Breast cancer is the most common cancer among women worldwide, and dietary factors may play a role in its prevention. While research on the association between tomato consumption and breast cancer risk is ongoing, some studies have suggested a potential protective effect of lycopene against breast cancer development. Lycopene's antioxidant properties help protect breast tissue from oxidative damage and reduce inflammation, which are both implicated in breast cancer progression.

7.6 Conclusion:

Tomatoes, rich in the powerful antioxidant lycopene, offer promising potential in cancer prevention. From reducing the risk of prostate cancer in men to protecting against lung, stomach, and breast cancer, tomatoes' anticancer properties are supported by a growing body of scientific evidence. By incorporating tomatoes and lycopene-rich foods into a balanced diet, individuals can take proactive steps to reduce their risk of cancer and promote overall health and well-being.

11

Chapter 8: Tomatoes for Eye Health

The eyes are often referred to as the windows to the soul, and maintaining good eye health is essential for overall well-being. In this chapter, we'll explore the role of tomatoes in promoting eye health and protecting against age-related vision problems.

8.1 Vision Nutrients in Tomatoes:

Tomatoes are rich in nutrients that are crucial for maintaining healthy eyesight, including vitamin C, vitamin E, beta-carotene, lutein, and zeaxanthin. These nutrients have antioxidant properties that help protect the eyes from oxidative damage caused by exposure to harmful ultraviolet (UV) rays, environmental pollutants, and free radicals. Additionally, these nutrients support the health and function of the retina, the light-sensitive tissue at the back of the eye responsible for transmitting visual information to the brain.

8.2 Lutein and Zeaxanthin:

Lutein and zeaxanthin are carotenoid pigments found in high concentrations in the macula, a small area in the center of the retina responsible for central vision and visual acuity. These pigments act as natural filters, absorbing harmful blue light and protecting the macula from oxidative damage. Studies have shown that higher dietary intake of lutein and zeaxanthin is associated with a reduced risk of age-related macular degeneration (AMD), a leading cause of vision loss in older adults. Tomatoes, particularly cooked or processed tomatoes, are a rich source of lutein and zeaxanthin, making them valuable for maintaining macular health.

8.3 Protection Against Cataracts:

Cataracts are a common age-related eye condition characterized by clouding of the lens, which can lead to blurry vision and eventually blindness if left untreated. Oxidative stress and inflammation are believed to play a role in the development of cataracts. The antioxidants found in tomatoes, including vitamin C, vitamin E, and lycopene, help neutralize free radicals and reduce inflammation, thereby protecting against cataract formation. Regular consumption of tomatoes and other antioxidant-rich foods may help reduce the risk of cataracts and preserve clear vision.

8.4 Glaucoma Prevention:

Glaucoma is a group of eye conditions characterized by damage to the optic nerve, often associated with increased intraocular pressure (IOP). While the exact cause of glaucoma is not fully understood, oxidative stress and impaired blood flow to the optic nerve are believed to contribute to its development. The antioxidants in tomatoes help improve blood flow to the optic nerve and protect against oxidative damage, potentially reducing the risk of glaucoma. While tomatoes alone may not prevent or treat glaucoma, incorporating them into a diet rich in other antioxidant-rich foods may help support overall eye health and reduce the risk of glaucoma-related complications.

8.5 Conclusion:

Tomatoes are not only delicious additions to meals but also valuable allies in promoting eye health and preventing age-related vision problems. From protecting against macular degeneration and cataracts to supporting overall ocular function, the nutrients, and antioxidants found in tomatoes offer a multitude of benefits for maintaining clear vision and healthy eyes. By incorporating tomatoes into your diet regularly, you can nourish your eyes and enjoy the many flavors and nutrients that nature's red treasure has to offer.

12

Chapter 9: Skin Benefits of Tomatoes

The skin is the body's largest organ, and maintaining its health and vitality is essential for overall well-being. In this chapter, we'll explore the numerous skin benefits of tomatoes and how incorporating them into your diet and skincare routine can help promote healthy, radiant skin.

9.1 Rich in Antioxidants:

Tomatoes are packed with antioxidants, including vitamin C, vitamin E, beta-carotene, and lycopene, which help protect the skin from damage caused by environmental pollutants, UV radiation, and free radicals. These antioxidants neutralize free radicals, preventing oxidative stress and reducing inflammation in the skin. By combatting oxidative stress and inflammation, tomatoes help maintain skin elasticity, reduce the appearance of wrinkles and fine lines, and promote a youthful complexion.

9.2 UV Protection:

Exposure to ultraviolet (UV) radiation from the sun can cause sunburn, premature aging, and an increased risk of skin cancer. The lycopene found in tomatoes acts as a natural sunscreen, absorbing UV radiation and protecting the skin from sun damage. While lycopene alone is not a substitute for sunscreen, incorporating tomatoes into your diet can provide additional protection against UV-induced skin damage and help maintain healthy skin.

9.3 Skin Hydration:

Tomatoes are composed primarily of water, making them an excellent source of hydration for the skin. When consumed as part of a balanced diet, the water content in tomatoes helps keep the skin hydrated from the inside out, reducing dryness, flakiness, and roughness. Additionally, applying tomato-based skincare products topically can help hydrate the skin and improve its moisture barrier function, resulting in soft, supple skin.

9.4 Acne Treatment:

Acne is a common skin condition characterized by clogged pores, inflammation, and the formation of pimples and blemishes. The salicylic acid found in tomatoes helps unclog pores and exfoliate dead skin cells, reducing the occurrence of acne breakouts. Additionally, the antioxidants and vitamins in tomatoes help reduce inflammation, soothe irritated skin, and promote healing, making tomatoes a valuable ingredient in natural acne treatments.

9.5 Brightening and Even Skin Tone:

The vitamin C and lycopene in tomatoes have skin-brightening properties that help reduce hyperpigmentation, dark spots, and uneven skin tone. Vitamin C inhibits the production of melanin, the pigment responsible for skin color, while lycopene helps fade existing dark spots and prevent the formation of new ones. Regular consumption of tomatoes and topical application of tomato-based skincare products can help promote a brighter, more even complexion.

9.6 Conclusion:

Tomatoes offer a myriad of skin benefits, from protecting against UV damage and reducing inflammation to hydrating the skin and promoting a youthful, radiant complexion. Whether consumed as part of a healthy diet or applied topically in skincare products, tomatoes can help nourish and rejuvenate the skin, revealing its natural beauty. By incorporating tomatoes into your daily routine, you can harness the power of nature's red treasure and achieve healthy, glowing skin from the inside out.

13

Chapter 10: Tomatoes and Digestive Health

Chapter 10: Tomatoes and Digestive Health

The digestive system plays a crucial role in overall health, and maintaining its proper function is essential for nutrient absorption, waste elimination, and overall well-being. In this chapter, we'll explore the impact of tomatoes on digestive health and how they can support a healthy gastrointestinal tract.

10.1 Fiber Content:

Tomatoes are an excellent source of dietary fiber, which is essential for maintaining a healthy digestive system. Fiber helps promote regular bowel movements by adding bulk to the stool and stimulating peristalsis, the rhythmic contractions of the intestinal muscles that propel food through the digestive tract. By promoting regularity, fiber helps prevent constipation, bloating, and other digestive discomforts, ensuring smooth and efficient digestion.

10.2 Improved Gut Microbiota:

The gut microbiota, composed of trillions of beneficial bacteria, plays a crucial role in digestion, nutrient absorption, and immune function. Emerging research suggests that tomatoes, particularly those rich in fiber and antioxidants, may help support a diverse and healthy gut microbiota. The fiber in tomatoes serves as a prebiotic, providing fuel for beneficial gut bacteria and promoting their growth and proliferation. Additionally, the antioxidants in tomatoes help reduce inflammation in the gut and support a balanced microbial ecosystem, contributing to overall digestive health.

10.3 Anti-inflammatory Effects:

Chronic inflammation in the digestive tract can lead to various gastrointestinal conditions, including inflammatory bowel disease (IBD), Crohn's disease, and ulcerative colitis. The antioxidants and phytonutrients found in tomatoes, particularly lycopene and vitamin C, possess anti-inflammatory properties that help reduce inflammation in the gut lining and alleviate symptoms associated with digestive disorders. By combating inflammation, tomatoes help promote a healthy digestive environment and support optimal gastrointestinal function.

10.4 Protection Against Gastric Ulcers:

Gastric ulcers, also known as peptic ulcers, are open sores that develop on the lining of the stomach or small intestine, often due to infection with the bacterium Helicobacter pylori or prolonged use of nonsteroidal anti-inflammatory drugs (NSAIDs). Studies have shown that the antioxidants and phytochemicals in tomatoes, including vitamin C, vitamin E, and flavonoids, help protect against gastric ulcers by reducing oxidative stress, inhibiting the growth of H. pylori bacteria, and promoting mucosal healing in the digestive tract. By incorporating tomatoes into your diet, you can help protect against gastric ulcers and maintain a healthy stomach lining.

10.5 Conclusion:

Tomatoes offer numerous benefits for digestive health, from promoting regularity and supporting healthy gut microbiota to reducing inflammation and protecting against gastric ulcers. Whether consumed fresh, cooked, or processed into sauces and soups, tomatoes provide valuable nutrients and phytochemicals that nourish the digestive system and promote optimal gastrointestinal function. By incorporating tomatoes into your daily diet, you can enjoy their delicious flavor while reaping the digestive benefits of nature's red treasure.

14

Chapter 11: Tomatoes: A Natural Anti-inflammatory

Inflammation is the body's natural response to injury, infection, or irritation, but chronic inflammation can lead to various health problems, including heart disease, cancer, and autoimmune disorders. In this chapter, we'll explore how tomatoes serve as a natural anti-inflammatory food and contribute to reducing inflammation throughout the body.

11.1 Phytonutrients and Antioxidants:

Tomatoes are rich in phytonutrients and antioxidants that possess potent anti-inflammatory properties. These include lycopene, vitamin C, vitamin E, beta-carotene, and various flavonoids and polyphenols. These compounds help neutralize free radicals and reduce oxidative stress, which are key contributors to inflammation. By scavenging free radicals and inhibiting inflammatory pathways, tomatoes help modulate the body's inflammatory response and promote overall health and well-being.

11.2 Reduction of Systemic Inflammation:

Chronic systemic inflammation is linked to the development of numerous chronic diseases, including cardiovascular disease, diabetes, arthritis, and Alzheimer's disease. Studies have shown that regular consumption of tomatoes and tomato-based products is associated with reduced levels of inflammatory markers in the blood, such as C-reactive protein (CRP) and interleukin-6 (IL-6). The anti-inflammatory effects of tomatoes help lower systemic inflammation and reduce the risk of chronic disease development.

11.3 Joint Health and Arthritis:

Arthritis is a common inflammatory condition characterized by pain, stiffness, and swelling in the joints. The anti-inflammatory properties of tomatoes can help alleviate symptoms associated with arthritis and support joint health. Lycopene, in particular, has been shown to reduce the production of inflammatory cytokines and enzymes that contribute to joint inflammation and cartilage degradation. By incorporating tomatoes into their diet, individuals with arthritis may experience relief from pain and improved joint function.

11.4 Skin Conditions:

Inflammatory skin conditions such as acne, eczema, and psoriasis can be exacerbated by chronic inflammation and oxidative stress. The antioxidants and phytonutrients in tomatoes help reduce inflammation in the skin and promote healing of damaged tissues. Additionally, the vitamin C in tomatoes supports collagen production, which is essential for maintaining skin elasticity and preventing wrinkles. Topical application of tomato-based skincare products may help soothe irritated skin and reduce redness and inflammation associated with inflammatory skin conditions.

11.5 Respiratory Health:

Inflammation in the respiratory tract can contribute to conditions such as asthma, bronchitis, and chronic obstructive pulmonary disease (COPD). The anti-inflammatory properties of tomatoes help reduce inflammation in the airways and improve respiratory function. Studies have shown that lycopene and other antioxidants in tomatoes may help alleviate symptoms of asthma and reduce the frequency and severity of asthma attacks. By incorporating tomatoes into their diet, individuals with respiratory conditions may experience improved lung function and respiratory health.

11.6 Conclusion:

Tomatoes are not only delicious and versatile but also powerful anti-inflammatory foods that offer numerous health benefits. From reducing systemic inflammation and supporting joint health to alleviating skin conditions and improving respiratory function, tomatoes play a valuable role in promoting overall health and well-being. By incorporating tomatoes into your diet regularly, whether fresh, cooked, or in the form of sauces and soups, you can harness the anti-inflammatory properties of nature's red treasure and enjoy its many health-promoting   effects.

15

Chapter 12: Tomatoes and Bone Health

While tomatoes are often celebrated for their vibrant color and delicious flavor, their potential benefits for bone health are less commonly known. In this chapter, we'll explore the role of tomatoes in supporting bone health and preventing osteoporosis and other bone-related conditions.

12.1 Nutrients for Bone Health:

Tomatoes contain several key nutrients that are essential for maintaining strong and healthy bones. These include vitamin K, potassium, calcium, and magnesium, all of which play critical roles in bone metabolism and mineralization. Vitamin K is particularly important for bone health, as it helps regulate calcium levels in the bones and promotes the activity of osteocalcin, a protein involved in bone formation. Potassium, calcium, and magnesium also contribute to bone density and strength, helping to prevent fractures and osteoporosis.

12.2 Vitamin K:

Vitamin K is a fat-soluble vitamin that plays a crucial role in bone metabolism and mineralization. It is involved in the synthesis of osteocalcin, a protein that binds calcium and helps incorporate it into the bone matrix. Adequate vitamin K intake has been associated with higher bone mineral density and reduced risk of fractures and osteoporosis. Tomatoes are a good source of vitamin K, particularly when consumed as part of a balanced diet that includes other vitamin K-rich foods like leafy greens, broccoli, and Brussels sprouts.

12.3 Potassium:

Potassium is an essential mineral that helps maintain electrolyte balance, regulate blood pressure, and support muscle function. Emerging research suggests that potassium may also play a role in bone health by neutralizing acids in the body and preserving calcium stores in the bones. Low potassium intake has been associated with increased urinary calcium excretion and higher risk of osteoporosis. Tomatoes are a rich source of potassium, with one medium-sized tomato providing approximately 10% of the daily recommended intake.

12.4 Lycopene and Bone Health:

While lycopene is best known for its antioxidant properties, emerging evidence suggests that it may also benefit bone health. Studies have shown that lycopene supplementation can improve bone mineral density and reduce bone resorption, the process by which old bone tissue is broken down and replaced by new bone. Additionally, lycopene's anti-inflammatory effects may help reduce oxidative stress and inflammation in the bones, further supporting bone health and preventing age-related bone loss.

12.5 Phytochemicals and Bone Protection:

In addition to vitamin K, potassium, and lycopene, tomatoes contain a variety of phytochemicals, including flavonoids and carotenoids, which may offer protection against bone-related conditions. Some studies have suggested that certain phytochemicals found in tomatoes, such as quercetin and naringenin, may help inhibit bone resorption and promote bone formation. While more research is needed to fully understand the mechanisms underlying the bone-protective effects of phytochemicals in tomatoes, incorporating tomatoes into a balanced diet can certainly contribute to overall bone health.

12.6 Conclusion:

Tomatoes are not only delicious and nutritious but also beneficial for bone health. Packed with vitamin K, potassium, lycopene, and other phytochemicals, tomatoes offer a natural way to support bone density, strength, and integrity. By incorporating tomatoes into your diet regularly and combining them with other bone-healthy foods and lifestyle habits, you can help maintain strong and resilient bones throughout life.

16

Chapter 13: Tomatoes in Weight Management

In the pursuit of a healthy weight, dietary choices play a crucial role. Tomatoes, with their low-calorie content, high water content, and an array of nutrients, can be valuable allies in weight management. In this chapter, we'll explore how tomatoes can support weight loss and maintenance.

13.1 Low Calorie and High Water Content:

Tomatoes are naturally low in calories, making them an excellent choice for those looking to manage their weight. One medium-sized tomato contains only about 25 calories, allowing you to enjoy its delicious flavor without consuming excess calories. Additionally, tomatoes have a high water content, which helps promote feelings of fullness and satiety. Including tomatoes in meals and snacks can help you stay satisfied while keeping your calorie intake in check, making them a valuable addition to a weight loss or weight maintenance plan.

13.2 Fiber for Satiety:

Fiber is another key component of tomatoes that supports weight management. Tomatoes contain both soluble and insoluble fiber, which help promote feelings of fullness and prevent overeating. Soluble fiber forms a gel-like substance in the stomach, slowing down digestion and delaying the emptying of the stomach, which helps keep you feeling full for longer. Insoluble fiber adds bulk to the stool and promotes regular bowel movements, preventing constipation and bloating. By including tomatoes in your diet, you can increase your fiber intake and support your weight loss goals.

13.3 Nutrient Density:

Despite being low in calories, tomatoes are packed with essential nutrients that are important for overall health and well-being. They are rich in vitamins A, C, and K, as well as potassium, manganese, and folate. These nutrients support various bodily functions, including immune function, skin health, and bone health, ensuring that you receive adequate nutrition while managing your weight. By choosing nutrient-dense foods like tomatoes, you can optimize your diet for both weight loss and overall health.

13.4 Versatile and Flavorful:

One of the advantages of tomatoes in weight management is their versatility and flavor. Tomatoes can be incorporated into a wide variety of dishes, including salads, soups, sandwiches, wraps, and stir-fries. They can also be eaten raw as a snack or appetizer, or cooked into sauces, salsas, and marinades. The versatility of tomatoes allows you to experiment with different recipes and meal ideas, keeping your meals exciting and satisfying while supporting your weight management goals.

13.5 Conclusion:

Tomatoes are an excellent addition to any weight management plan, thanks to their low-calorie content, high water and fiber content, and nutrient density. By including tomatoes in your meals and snacks, you can increase feelings of fullness, satisfy your taste buds, and ensure that you receive essential nutrients while managing your weight. Whether enjoyed fresh, cooked or in the form of sauces and soups, tomatoes offer a delicious and nutritious way to support your weight loss or weight maintenance journey.

17

Chapter 14: Tomatoes and Brain Health

The brain is arguably the most vital organ in the body, responsible for controlling thoughts, emotions, movements, and vital functions. Maintaining optimal brain health is essential for overall well-being and cognitive function. In this chapter, we'll explore the fascinating connection between tomatoes and brain health, uncovering the potential benefits of this red treasure for the mind.

14.1 Antioxidants and Neuroprotection:

Tomatoes are rich in antioxidants, including vitamin C, vitamin E, and lycopene, which play crucial roles in protecting the brain from oxidative stress and damage. Oxidative stress is implicated in the development of neurodegenerative diseases such as Alzheimer's and Parkinson's disease. The antioxidants in tomatoes help neutralize free radicals and reduce inflammation in the brain, thereby protecting neurons and supporting overall brain health.

14.2 Lycopene and Cognitive Function:

Lycopene, the vibrant red pigment in tomatoes, has garnered attention for its potential role in preserving cognitive function and reducing the risk of neurodegenerative diseases. Studies have shown that lycopene supplementation may improve cognitive performance and memory in older adults. Additionally, lycopene's antioxidant and anti-inflammatory properties help protect against the oxidative damage and neuroinflammation associated with Alzheimer's and Parkinson's disease, potentially slowing the progression of these debilitating conditions.

14.3 Improved Blood Flow to the Brain:

Proper blood flow to the brain is essential for delivering oxygen and nutrients and removing metabolic waste products. Reduced blood flow to the brain is associated with cognitive decline and an increased risk of neurodegenerative diseases. The nitric oxide-boosting properties of certain compounds in tomatoes, such as nitrates and antioxidants, help promote vasodilation and improve blood flow to the brain. By enhancing cerebral blood flow, tomatoes support brain function and may reduce the risk of cognitive impairment.

14.4 Neuroprotective Effects of Potassium:

Tomatoes are a good source of potassium, a mineral that plays a vital role in maintaining healthy brain function. Potassium helps regulate nerve transmission, muscle contraction, and fluid balance in the body, all of which are essential for proper brain function. Adequate potassium intake has been associated with improved cognitive performance and reduced risk of stroke, a leading cause of cognitive impairment and dementia. Including potassium-rich foods like tomatoes in your diet can help support brain health and cognitive function.

14.5 Mental Well-being:

In addition to protecting against neurodegenerative diseases, tomatoes may also support mental well-being and mood. Certain nutrients in tomatoes, such as vitamin C and folate, are involved in the synthesis of neurotransmitters like serotonin and dopamine, which play key roles in regulating mood and emotions. Furthermore, the anti-inflammatory properties of tomatoes help reduce inflammation in the brain, which has been linked to depression and anxiety. By nourishing the brain with nutrient-rich foods like tomatoes, you can support mental health and cognitive function.

14.6 Conclusion:

Tomatoes offer a wealth of benefits for brain health, from protecting against neurodegenerative diseases to supporting cognitive function and mental well-being. Packed with antioxidants, lycopene, potassium, and other essential nutrients, tomatoes provide valuable support for the brain's structure and function. By incorporating tomatoes into your diet regularly, whether fresh, cooked, or in the form of sauces and soups, you can nourish your brain and unlock the potential of nature's red treasure for optimal brain health and cognitive   vitality.

18

Chapter 15: Tomatoes for Glowing Hair

While tomatoes are renowned for their culinary versatility and health benefits, their potential for enhancing hair health is often overlooked. In this chapter, we'll explore the surprising ways in which tomatoes can contribute to achieving lustrous, glowing hair.

15.1 Rich in Vitamins and Minerals:

Tomatoes are packed with essential vitamins and minerals that are vital for hair health. These include vitamin A, vitamin C, vitamin E, biotin, and various B vitamins such as folate, thiamine, and riboflavin. These nutrients play key roles in promoting scalp health, supporting hair growth, and maintaining the strength and luster of hair strands. By incorporating tomatoes into your diet, you can provide your hair with the nourishment it needs to shine from within.

15.2 Promotes Scalp Health:

A healthy scalp is the foundation for healthy hair growth, and tomatoes can help promote scalp health in several ways. The vitamin C and antioxidants in tomatoes help protect the scalp from oxidative stress and environmental damage, preventing scalp irritation and inflammation. Additionally, the acidic nature of tomatoes helps balance the pH level of the scalp, reducing oiliness and preventing dandruff. Including tomatoes in your diet or using tomato-based hair treatments can help keep your scalp healthy and flake-free.

15.3 Strengthens Hair Strands:

The vitamins and minerals found in tomatoes, particularly vitamin A, vitamin E, and biotin, play crucial roles in strengthening hair strands and preventing breakage and split ends. Vitamin A promotes the production of sebum, a natural oil that moisturizes the scalp and keeps hair strands hydrated and supple. Vitamin E acts as a powerful antioxidant, protecting hair follicles from damage caused by free radicals and environmental stressors. Biotin, also known as vitamin B7, supports keratin production, the protein that forms the structure of hair, nails, and skin. Including tomatoes in your diet can help fortify your hair strands from within, promoting resilience and shine.

15.4 Stimulates Hair Growth:

For those looking to promote hair growth and combat hair loss, tomatoes offer a natural solution. The vitamins and antioxidants in tomatoes help improve blood circulation to the scalp, delivering essential nutrients and oxygen to the hair follicles and stimulating hair growth. Additionally, the lycopene in tomatoes has been shown to inhibit the activity of 5-alpha reductase, an enzyme involved in the conversion of testosterone to dihydrotestosterone (DHT), a hormone linked to hair loss. By incorporating tomatoes into your diet or using tomato-based hair treatments, you can encourage healthy hair growth and maintain a full, voluminous mane.

15.5 Adds Shine and Luster:

The acidic nature of tomatoes helps seal the hair cuticle, resulting in smoother, shinier hair strands. The vitamins and antioxidants in tomatoes nourish the hair from the inside out, enhancing its natural luster and radiance. Additionally, the high water content of tomatoes helps hydrate the hair strands, preventing dryness and frizz. Whether consumed as part of a balanced diet or applied topically as a hair mask or rinse, tomatoes can help you achieve glossy, healthy-looking hair that shines with vitality.

15.6 Conclusion:

Tomatoes offer a multitude of benefits for achieving glowing, healthy hair, thanks to their rich nutrient profile and unique properties. From promoting scalp health and strengthening hair strands to stimulating hair growth and adding shine, tomatoes provide a natural and effective solution for hair care. By incorporating tomatoes into your diet and skincare routine, you can harness the power of nature's red treasure to unlock the full potential of your hair and achieve the radiant locks you've always desired.

19

Chapter 16: Tomatoes in Skincare

Tomatoes, with their vibrant color and juicy texture, are not only a delightful addition to culinary creations but also hold remarkable potential in skincare. In this chapter, we'll delve into the myriad benefits of tomatoes for the skin and explore how incorporating them into your skincare routine can help unlock nature's red treasure for a radiant complexion.

16.1 Antioxidant Powerhouse:

Tomatoes are rich in antioxidants, including vitamin C, vitamin E, beta-carotene, and lycopene, which help protect the skin from oxidative damage caused by free radicals and environmental stressors. These antioxidants neutralize harmful free radicals, preventing premature aging, reducing inflammation, and promoting overall skin health. Incorporating tomatoes into your skincare routine can help defend against environmental aggressors and keep your skin looking youthful and radiant.

16.2 Brightens and Evens Skin Tone:

The vitamin C and lycopene in tomatoes have skin-brightening properties that help reduce hyperpigmentation, dark spots, and uneven skin tone. Vitamin C inhibits the production of melanin, the pigment responsible for skin color, while lycopene helps fade existing dark spots and prevent the formation of new ones. Regular use of tomato-based skincare products or homemade tomato masks can help promote a brighter, more even complexion, revealing the natural beauty of your skin.

16.3 Controls Oiliness and Acne:

Tomatoes possess astringent properties that help tighten pores and regulate sebum production, making them effective for controlling oiliness and preventing acne breakouts. The natural acids in tomatoes help balance the skin's pH level, reducing excess oil production and preventing clogged pores. Additionally, the antioxidants and vitamins in tomatoes help reduce inflammation and soothe irritated skin, making them beneficial for acne-prone skin. Using tomato-based toners or cleansers can help purify the skin and keep acne at bay.

16.4 Hydrates and Nourishes:

The high water content of tomatoes makes them excellent hydrating agents for the skin. Tomatoes help replenish moisture, leaving the skin soft, supple, and hydrated. Additionally, the vitamins and minerals in tomatoes nourish the skin, providing essential nutrients that promote overall skin health. Applying tomato-based face masks or serums can help quench thirsty skin and restore its natural radiance.

16.5 Exfoliates and Renews:

Tomatoes contain natural acids, such as citric acid and malic acid, which gently exfoliate the skin, removing dead skin cells and promoting cell turnover. Regular exfoliation with tomato-based products helps reveal fresh, smooth skin and improves the absorption of skincare products. Additionally, the antioxidants in tomatoes help repair and rejuvenate the skin, reducing the appearance of fine lines, wrinkles, and other signs of aging.

16.6 Soothes Sunburns:

The cooling and anti-inflammatory properties of tomatoes make them effective for soothing sunburns and reducing redness and irritation. The vitamins and antioxidants in tomatoes help promote skin healing and repair damaged cells, providing relief from sunburn symptoms. Applying freshly sliced tomatoes or tomato-based compresses to sunburned skin can help alleviate discomfort and speed up the recovery process.

16.7 Conclusion:

Tomatoes are versatile skincare ingredients that offer a multitude of benefits for the skin, from brightening and evening skin tone to controlling oiliness, hydrating, and nourishing. Whether used in homemade masks, serums, toners, or commercial skin care products, tomatoes can help you achieve a radiant complexion and unleash the natural beauty of your skin. By incorporating tomatoes into your skincare routine, you can harness the power of nature's red treasure and enjoy healthy, glowing skin year-round.

20

Chapter 17: Cooking with Tomatoes: Delicious and Nutritious Recipes from Around the World

Tomatoes are a versatile ingredient that features prominently in cuisines from various cultures around the world. From Mediterranean dishes to Latin American specialties, tomatoes add depth of flavor, vibrant color, and nutritional benefits to a wide range of recipes. In this chapter, we'll explore some delicious and nutritious tomato-based recipes from different culinary traditions.

17.1 Italian Caprese Salad:

Originating from Italy, Caprese salad is a classic dish that celebrates the simplicity and freshness of tomatoes. To make this flavorful salad, slice ripe tomatoes and fresh mozzarella cheese and arrange them on a plate. Drizzle with extra-virgin olive oil, sprinkle with chopped fresh basil leaves, and season with salt and pepper to taste. Serve as a refreshing appetizer or side dish, and enjoy the harmony of flavors and textures.

17.2 Spanish Gazpacho:

Gazpacho is a chilled tomato soup that hails from Spain and is perfect for hot summer days. To prepare gazpacho, blend ripe tomatoes, cucumber, bell peppers, onions, garlic, and stale bread until smooth. Season with olive oil, vinegar, salt, and pepper, and chill in the refrigerator for several hours to allow the flavors to meld. Serve cold with a garnish of chopped vegetables and a drizzle of olive oil for a refreshing and nutritious meal.

17.3 Indian Tomato Curry (Tamatar Ki Sabzi):

In Indian cuisine, tomatoes are often used as a base for flavorful curries and sauces. To make tomato curry, heat oil in a pan and sauté onions, garlic, ginger, and spices such as cumin, coriander, turmeric, and chili powder. Add chopped tomatoes and cook until they break down and form a thick sauce. Finish with a splash of coconut milk or cream for richness, and garnish with fresh cilantro. Serve with rice or flatbread for a satisfying and aromatic meal.

17.4 Mexican Salsa Fresca:

Salsa fresca, also known as pico de gallo, is a fresh and zesty salsa that is popular in Mexican cuisine. To make salsa fresca, diced ripe tomatoes, onions, jalapeños, cilantro, and lime juice. Season with salt and pepper to taste, and stir to combine. Serve as a topping for tacos, quesadillas, or grilled meats, or enjoy with tortilla chips as a refreshing snack. Salsa Fresca adds a burst of flavor and brightness to any dish.

17.5 Greek Spanakopita:

Spanakopita is a traditional Greek dish made with layers of phyllo pastry filled with spinach, feta cheese, and tomatoes. To make spanakopita, sauté spinach, onions, garlic, and dill until wilted, then mix with crumbled feta cheese and diced tomatoes. Layer the spinach mixture between sheets of phyllo pastry, brushing each layer with olive oil, and bake until golden and crispy. Serve warm as a savory appetizer or side dish, and savor the delicious combination of flavors.

17.6 Thai Green Papaya Salad (Som Tam):

Som Tam is a vibrant and spicy salad from Thailand that features green papaya, tomatoes, and a tangy dressing. To make Som Tam, shred green papaya and toss with diced tomatoes, green beans, peanuts, and Thai chili peppers. Dress with a mixture of lime juice, fish sauce, palm sugar, and garlic, and toss to combine. Serve as a refreshing and invigorating salad, and enjoy the bold flavors of Thai cuisine.

17.7 Conclusion:

Tomatoes are a versatile and nutritious ingredient that adds flavor, color, and health benefits to a wide range of dishes from around the world. Whether incorporated into salads, soups, curries, salsas, or savory pies, tomatoes are sure to elevate any meal with their vibrant taste and nutritional value. Experiment with these delicious recipes and discover the culinary delights of tomatoes from different culinary traditions.

21

Chapter 18: Preserving Tomatoes: From Canning to Sun-Drying

Tomatoes are a seasonal delight, abundant during the summer months when they're at their ripest and most flavorful. However, with proper preservation techniques, you can enjoy the delicious taste of tomatoes year-round. In this chapter, we'll explore various methods of preserving tomatoes, from canning to sun-drying, allowing you to savor nature's red treasure long after the harvest season ends.

18.1 Canning Tomatoes:

Canning is one of the most popular methods of preserving tomatoes, allowing you to store them for an extended period without losing their flavor or nutritional value. To can tomatoes, start by washing and sterilizing canning jars and lids. Blanch the tomatoes in boiling water for a few minutes, then transfer them to the jars, leaving a half-inch of headspace. Add lemon juice or citric acid to acidify the tomatoes and prevent spoilage. Process the jars in a boiling water bath for the recommended time based on altitude and jar size. Once cooled, store the canned tomatoes in a cool, dark place for up to a year, enjoying their delicious taste in sauces, soups, and stews throughout the year.

18.2 Freezing Tomatoes:

Freezing is another convenient method of preserving tomatoes, requiring minimal effort and equipment. To freeze tomatoes, start by washing and drying them thoroughly. Remove any stems and cores, then cut the tomatoes into desired sizes or leave them whole, depending on your preference. Arrange the tomatoes in a single layer on a baking sheet and freeze until firm. Once frozen, transfer the tomatoes to freezer-safe bags or containers, removing as much air as possible before sealing. Store the frozen tomatoes in the freezer for up to six months, using them in sauces, salsas, and other dishes straight from the freezer for a burst of fresh tomato flavor.

18.3 Sun-Drying Tomatoes:

Sun-drying is a traditional method of preserving tomatoes that intensifies their flavor and creates deliciously sweet and chewy dried tomatoes. To sun-dry tomatoes, start by slicing them into halves or quarters and removing the seeds and excess moisture. Arrange the tomato slices on a drying rack or mesh screen in a sunny, well-ventilated area. Sprinkle the tomatoes with salt and herbs, such as oregano or basil, for added flavor. Allow the tomatoes to dry in the sun for several days, turning them occasionally to ensure even drying. Once the tomatoes are dried to your desired consistency, store them in airtight containers or jars with olive oil for up to six months, using them in salads, pasta dishes, and antipasto platters for a burst of sun-ripened tomato flavor.

18.4 Tomato Paste and Sauce:

Tomato paste and sauce are convenient pantry staples that add depth of flavor and richness to a wide range of dishes. To make tomato paste, start by blanching and peeling ripe tomatoes, then puree them in a blender or food processor until smooth. Cook the tomato puree in a saucepan over low heat, stirring occasionally, until it thickens and reduces by half. Transfer the thickened tomato paste to sterilized jars and process in a boiling water bath for long-term storage. For tomato sauce, follow a similar process, adding onions, garlic, herbs, and spices to the pureed tomatoes before cooking them down into a thick, flavorful sauce. Store the tomato paste and sauce in a cool, dark place for up to a year, enjoying their rich taste in pasta dishes, pizzas, and soups whenever you need a taste of summer.

18.5 Conclusion:

Preserving tomatoes allows you to enjoy the delicious taste of nature's red treasure year-round, whether canned, frozen, sun-dried, or transformed into paste and sauce. By following these preservation methods, you can savor the flavor and nutritional benefits of tomatoes in your favorite recipes, even when they're out of season. Experiment with different preservation techniques and discover the joy of preserving tomatoes for delicious meals and culinary delights throughout the year.

22

Chapter 19: Tomatoes in Popular Culture

Tomatoes have left an indelible mark on popular culture, appearing in various forms across literature, art, film, music, and even folklore. From their symbolic significance to their portrayal in media, tomatoes have become iconic symbols of vitality, love, and culinary delight. In this chapter, we'll explore the diverse ways in which tomatoes have permeated popular culture and captured the imagination of people around the world.

19.1 Cultural Symbolism:

Throughout history, tomatoes have held symbolic significance in different cultures. In some societies, tomatoes are associated with love and passion, often featuring prominently in romantic gestures and expressions of affection. In others, tomatoes symbolize vitality, health, and abundance, celebrated in festivals and rituals honoring the harvest season. Additionally, tomatoes have been used symbolically in literature and art to represent themes of growth, transformation, and the cycle of life.

19.2 Culinary Inspiration:

Tomatoes have long been celebrated in the culinary world, inspiring chefs and home cooks alike to create a myriad of delicious dishes. From classic Italian pasta sauces to Mexican salsas and Greek salads, tomatoes are a versatile ingredient that adds depth of flavor and vibrant color to countless recipes. Their popularity in cuisine has led to the creation of iconic dishes and culinary traditions that celebrate the rich taste and nutritional benefits of tomatoes.

19.3 Advertising and Marketing:

Tomatoes have also played a prominent role in advertising and marketing, featured in commercials, print ads, and product packaging to promote various food and beverage products. Their bright red color and juicy texture make them visually appealing and instantly recognizable, capturing the attention of consumers and enticing them to purchase tomato-based products. Whether showcased in advertisements for ketchup, pasta sauce, or tomato juice, tomatoes have become synonymous with freshness, flavor, and quality.

19.4 Film and Television:

Tomatoes have made cameo appearances in numerous films and television shows, often as a symbol of comfort, nostalgia, or comedic effect. Whether depicted in scenes of family dinners, cooking competitions, or romantic encounters, tomatoes evoke a sense of warmth and familiarity that resonates with audiences. Additionally, tomatoes have been featured in documentaries and cooking shows that explore their cultural significance, nutritional benefits, and culinary versatility.

19.5 Literature and Art:

Tomatoes have been immortalized in literature and art, appearing in paintings, sculptures, poems, and novels that celebrate their beauty and significance. Artists have been inspired by the vibrant color and organic shape of tomatoes, incorporating them into still-life compositions and botanical illustrations. Similarly, writers have used tomatoes as metaphors for life, love, and the passage of time, weaving them into stories that evoke a sense of nostalgia and wonder.

19.6 Folklore and Mythology:

In some cultures, tomatoes have been surrounded by folklore and mythology, with stories and legends passed down through generations. These tales often attribute magical or mystical properties to tomatoes, portraying them as symbols of good fortune, protection, or fertility. Additionally, tomatoes have been incorporated into traditional rituals and ceremonies believed to bring luck, prosperity, and blessings to those who partake in them.

19.7 Conclusion:

Tomatoes hold a special place in popular culture, transcending geographical and cultural boundaries to become beloved symbols of vitality, love, and culinary delight. From their portrayal in literature, art, film, and television to their role in advertising, folklore, and mythology, tomatoes have captured the imagination of people around the world, leaving an enduring legacy that continues to inspire and delight. As we celebrate the rich cultural heritage of tomatoes, let us savor their delicious taste and appreciate the beauty and symbolism they bring to our lives.

23

Chapter 20: The Future of Tomatoes: Innovations and Sustainable Practices

As we look to the future, tomatoes hold promise as a sustainable and versatile crop that can help address global food security challenges while promoting environmental stewardship and innovation. In this chapter, we'll explore the exciting developments and sustainable practices shaping the future of tomatoes and the agricultural industry as a whole.

20.1 Vertical Farming:

Vertical farming is revolutionizing the way tomatoes are grown, offering a space-efficient and resource-efficient alternative to traditional agriculture. In vertical farms, tomatoes are cultivated in vertically stacked layers, utilizing hydroponic or aeroponic systems that deliver water, nutrients, and light directly to the plants. Vertical farming reduces the need for arable land, conserves water, and minimizes pesticide use, making it a sustainable solution for urban agriculture and food production in areas with limited space and resources.

20.2 Controlled Environment Agriculture (CEA):

Controlled environment agriculture involves growing tomatoes in controlled indoor environments, such as greenhouses or indoor vertical farms, where temperature, humidity, light, and nutrient levels can be precisely regulated. CEA allows for year-round cultivation of tomatoes, independent of seasonal variations and climatic conditions. By optimizing growing conditions and minimizing environmental stressors, CEA maximizes crop yields, enhances quality, and reduces resource inputs, contributing to more sustainable and resilient food production systems.

20.3 Precision Agriculture:

Precision agriculture employs advanced technologies, such as GPS, drones, sensors, and data analytics, to optimize resource management and decision-making in tomato cultivation. By collecting real-time data on soil conditions, weather patterns, crop health, and pest infestations, precision agriculture enables farmers to make informed choices and implement targeted interventions that minimize inputs and maximize yields. From precision irrigation and fertilization to integrated pest management and crop monitoring, precision agriculture enhances efficiency, productivity, and sustainability in tomato production.

20.4 Genetic Innovation:

Advancements in genetic engineering and breeding techniques are unlocking new possibilities for enhancing the flavor, nutritional content, and resilience of tomatoes. Researchers are developing genetically modified tomatoes with improved traits, such as disease resistance, drought tolerance, and shelf life, to address key challenges facing tomato growers. Additionally, efforts are underway to enhance the nutritional profile of tomatoes by increasing levels of vitamins, antioxidants, and other beneficial compounds, further promoting human health and well-being.

20.5 Sustainable Practices:

In response to growing concerns about environmental degradation and climate change, tomato producers are adopting sustainable farming practices that minimize environmental impact and promote ecosystem health. These practices include organic farming, crop rotation, cover cropping, conservation tillage, and integrated pest management, which reduce soil erosion, conserve water, promote biodiversity, and enhance soil fertility. By prioritizing sustainability and resilience, tomato growers can mitigate environmental risks and build a more sustainable future for agriculture.

20.6 Conclusion:

The future of tomatoes is bright, fueled by innovation, sustainability, and a commitment to addressing global food security challenges. From vertical farming and controlled environment agriculture to precision agriculture and genetic innovation, tomatoes are at the forefront of agricultural transformation. By embracing sustainable practices and harnessing the power of technology and innovation, we can ensure a bountiful harvest of tomatoes for generations to come, nourishing people and planet alike with nature's red treasure.

24

Chapter 24